Praise for
REACHING FOR THE MOON

Gentle, accessible, and written directly to the heart of young girls, this book introduces our daughters to the magic and mystery of womanhood, as well as the biological facts and practical information needed to lay the foundation for a healthy, lifelong relationship with their cycles. A must-read for all of our daughters!

Melia Keeton-Digby, author *The Heroines Club*, creator of The Mother-Daughter Nest

A beautiful, insightful book that every girl should have clenched to her heart. I recommend it to all mothers with daughters who are about to make the transition to womanhood. It is the most life affirming gift you could offer, a rite of passage.

Wendy Cook, founder, Mighty Girl Art™

*I absolutely **love** this book, it is a treasure. It really communicates with young girls how to honour their moon time, expressed in such a tender loving way.*

Donna Virgilio, 12Radio.com

Menstruation is a beautiful and powerful rite of passage that should add an exclamation point to girl's identity. Reaching for the Moon is a book that delivers the goods ... a book to be shared between mothers and daughters, honoring what it means to be a powerful and creative girl blossoming into a creative young woman. This book is filled with easy to understand gems of wisdom that uplift and honor girls, professing menarche as a special time in her life. I am grateful to Lucy Pearce for writing a book that is beautiful, gentle, wise and affirming, a treasure of a book that I have given my own daughters in celebration of their creative potential.

Becky Jaine, mother, writer, and joy and creativity activist at Joyfuel.org

A message of wonder, empowerment, magic and beauty in the shared secrets of our femininity... written to encourage girls to embrace their transition to womanhood in a knowledgeable, supported, loving way.

The Loving Parent.com

Lucy, what you are doing is a great service for women. Thank you for growing this consciousness as I see that our futures will be anchored with Red Tents for decades to come because we co-created a world where women honor themselves. For our daughters and their mothers, thank you.

ALisa Starkweather, founder, Red Tent Temple movement

Reaching for the Moon

Other books by the same author

Moon Time: harness the ever-changing energy of your menstrual cycle

The Rainbow Way: cultivating creativity in the midst of motherhood

Moods of Motherhood: the inner journey of mothering

Anthology Contributor

Earth Pathways Diary 2011–13

Note to Self: the Secret to Becoming your own Best Friend
Jo MacDonald (2012)

Musings on Mothering—La Leche League GB
mothersmilkbooks.com (2012)

Tiny Buddha's Guide to Loving Yourself
Hay House (2013)

Roots: Where Food Comes From and Where It Takes Us: A BlogHer Anthology (2013)

Also from Womancraft Publishing

The Heart of the Labyrinth—Nicole Schwab
Moods of Motherhood: the inner journey of mothering—Lucy H. Pearce

Moon Time: harness the ever-changing energy of your menstrual cycle—Lucy H. Pearce

Reaching for the Moon

OOO

Lucy H. Pearce

Womancraft Publishing

Reaching for the Moon

Cover art © Lucy Pearce
Cover design by Lucent Word
www.lucentword.com

Extended quotations used with the express permission of their authors.

The author is not a trained health practitioner. The information provided in this text should not be taken as personal medical or contraceptive advice or instruction. No action should be taken based solely on the contents of this text. Readers should consult appropriate health professionals on any matter relating to their health and well-being.

Second edition published by Womancraft Publishing, 2015
www.womancraftpublishing.com

ISBN: 978-1910559-086 (paperback)
ISBN: 978-1910559-093 (ebook)

OOO

For all our precious daughters,
may you know that you are loved more deeply than you can
possibly imagine.

OOO

At her first bleeding a woman meets her power.
During her bleeding years she practices it.
At menopause she becomes it.
Traditional Native American saying

CONTENTS

INTRODUCTION

Dearest girl,

This book is written for you, as you reach for the moon, and begin to change from girl to woman.

It contains the words that older women who love you very much want to pass on to you. Words just for girls.

In other cultures and other times, girls who were entering womanhood would be welcomed by their tribe. They would be told the secrets of womanhood, they would be tested for their strength and courage. They would be blessed and celebrated.

This book is our starting point. A way of celebrating your transition, and sharing our women's secrets with you. I hope that you will find, through the girls and women, boys and men that you love and trust, a circle of people to celebrate and support you as you grow and develop.

Each girl reading this will have different levels of knowledge and understanding. Each girl's body will be at a different stage. That is just as it should be. You may already know quite a lot of what is in this book. Or it may all be completely new to you and you may not be ready to hear it all now. That is just fine. Take what is right for you now. Think it over. And as you change more, or have more questions, you can come back to this book and the women you know with questions.

Please know that we remember how it is: the uncertainty of your changing body, changing feelings towards your parents, the pressures to decide who you will be and what you will do, the new feelings of intense love and passion, shifting friendships and wanting to fit in. We remember so clearly how our bodies changed before our eyes, and how those around us reacted. And we remember our first blood.

Surprise. Excitement. Shock. Relief. Sadness. Confusion. For some of us it came early, for others late, and a few never got it at all. Our bodies changes have a timing all of their own. They tell us secrets that we otherwise would not know.

We remember—though you may not see or feel our remembering. Sometimes we don't know quite the right words, or can't find quite the right time to say all the things we want to share with you. It can be hard to know where to start.

I wrote this book for my own daughters, and daughters of friends, to share the words that we sometimes find hard to say in real life.

What I want to say is this.

Your body. My body. Our bodies are incredible. But sometimes we aren't told this.

Throughout history, and even in the sacred books, women have been told that there is something wrong with them because they have women's bodies. Many of us have learned to be ashamed of our bodies and their natural functions. We have struggled to talk about them, we have not had the words.

For most of my generation, and our mothers and grandmothers before us, our changing bodies meant a time of awkwardness and embarrassment. Our women's cycles have often been a pain. And we have not been encouraged to talk about or respect our female bodies and their mysteries. In truth being a woman has been quite hard. Maybe you know this, maybe you have a sense of it. But that was our story. The future is yours.

We want to share with you how magnificent it can be to be a woman, how magical our bodies truly are. But to do that we have to have words, so we can share our stories, feelings and ideas.

I love words. Each has a different feeling and sound when you say it out loud or read it in your head. Each can make your body feel a different way. They can make you feel proud. Or make you feel yuck. When it comes to 'down there' there are nearly as many words as there are women!

But there are lots of girls and women who don't have any word that feels good for one of the most important parts of their bodies. It is of course your vagina … on the inside and your vulva on the outside. Others call it 'privates' or 'bits' or 'fanny' or 'front bum' or 'yoni'. *Yoni* means sacred space in Sanskrit—origin, source—it refers to the entire genital system. In India there are altars dedicated to the yoni, whole temples decorated with them!

What is yours? Whisper it quietly, I won't tell a soul! Shout it loud. Say it proud. It's your body … so name it! No need to giggle or be shy. Say it the same way you say 'elbow' or 'toe'.

And then as we travel further in, we have the magic cave, your uterus or womb. The hidden place where you came into being yourself and grew and grew. Your womb is the size of a pear on a normal day, the size of a grapefruit when you are menstruating and the size of a large watermelon when you're pregnant. A wonderful American midwife called Ina May Gaskin once said if men had a body part as incredible as a uterus, they would never stop boasting about it.

Most women have a womb—though a few girls are born without them. It's hidden away, up at the top of your vagina, you'll never see it, you can't really feel it … and yet it's a place where women's magic happens.

Introduction

This is the place where our story happens. It is a story of a womb. Your womb. Our wombs.

You and I are going on a journey together now, to a different time and place long ago where women's bodies were respected because they could make life. Once a month, all the women would gather—those bleeding, and those breastfeeding their babies, the pregnant women, the older women who were past their bleeding days, and the women who had bodies that had never bled. They would gather together to rest, talk, dream, laugh, cry, heal, share ideas and stories and support each other.

The red tent. A womb-like space where women come as their bodies do what most women's bodies naturally do once a month: lose the lining of their womb through a warm flow of blood.

These red tents are not just things of the past. They are our future too. In recent years they have been springing up all around the world in bedrooms and town halls, festivals and lounges. Women and girls come together and talk, and learn how awesome and precious their bodies are, and how important it is to care for them.

And that is where this book begins: in a place where only women can enter. A place that men guard and protect as sacred space. Perhaps it is a red tent of the past ... or the future. It is a place where you will feel safe and loved and accepted. Where women share their deepest secrets.

Come with me then, my love, into the red tent ...

THE SECRET OF THE RED TENT

A girl stands outside a red tent. Inside she hears the voices of her mother and aunts, their friends and neighbours. What do they talk about, when they are all alone? she wonders.

As a young girl she played outside, barely noticing their disappearance every month. But now, she finds herself drawn to this place of women, straining to hear the stories they share. Wanting so much to know what it is that makes them laugh like a vast tumbling river, or weep an ocean which stains their cheeks and leaves their eyes red-rimmed. What is it that these women do? These women whose lives seem both so boring and fascinating? Some who work in unknown places for hours each day, others who spend their lives changing nappies and cooking dinners. What is it that brings them together?

She creeps closer and pulls back the curtain. Peeping into the red tent she sees a beautiful woman dancing, her hips sliding, breasts full in a sparkling red top, hands flitting like butterflies as she shimmies around the candlelit room. The other women watch, eyes

7

sparkling like jewels, voices singing together, weaving a harmony—songs of water, women, the moon, birth and love. Then a bell is sounded, it echoes around the tent until only silence is left. And then after a while, one of the women begins to speak, gently at first, tears dripping down her cheeks, she tells of her sadness and pain. The women beside her hold her, stroking her hair as she weeps, and then almost like magic, her tears begin to dry and she is smiling once more.

Now another woman, older, with greying hair and beautiful smile lines, begins to speak. She tells a tale of passion and desire, that makes the listening girl blush— she has never heard women talking of lovers before, she has never really thought about how the grown-ups she knows share love with their bodies when their bedroom door is closed and the night is dark. She listens closer, straining to learn the secrets of love …

One of the women spots her face, peeping round the corner, and they laugh, beckoning her in. "We've been expecting you!" her mother says, "Dearest girl. I remember as if it was yesterday, when you grew in my belly, cradled in my womb. I will never forget the day of your birth, pushing you out of my body and into this world. Holding your precious tiny body in my arms. Feeding you from my breast. You will never remember those things, but I do.

"I remember the times when you were sick and I sat up with you at night, holding your hand when you were afraid. By our side you learnt to talk and walk, to read and write. We played dolls, made dens in the grass and climbed trees. And now, here you are, becoming a woman before our eyes. You, my love, are reaching for the moon!

"Come and take your place with us, it is time for you to learn some of our secrets.

- ○ The secret of your body
- ○ The secret of your blood
- ○ The secret of your fertility
- ○ The secret of the moon
- ○ The secret of self-care

"We have gifts to share with you:

- ○ The gift of celebration
- ○ The gift of intuition
- ○ The gift of sisterhood
- ○ The gift of herbs
- ○ The gift of the Crazy Woman

"At each stage of your birth into womanhood, there will be more secrets to share—as you come to first love, pregnancy, birth, motherhood and a deeper understanding of your cycles.

"But our task for now is to share with you the lessons of the moon. To let you know about the miracle in your belly, in your precious womb, which is coming alive right now. You cannot see it, you cannot touch it, but the magic in your womb will weave its way through your whole life: your feelings, your thoughts, your dreams.

"We will tell you stories of our own lives and answer your questions. We promise to do everything we can to support you as you reach for the moon.

"Each woman here is your sister. This is where we get to hear and know our own wisdom and that of all women. Here we get to find support for ourselves as we each walk our paths.

"You must honour this women's space and the responsibility of being allowed in.

- Respect the confidence of your sisters and their stories.

- Know that each has her own unique story full of darkness and light, if you will only listen.

- Do not judge or gossip about her—but take this chance to learn from her.

○ Learn to share your own story, to honour your
   own experience and share it with those who
   will honour it too."

A dark-eyed woman picks up a carved wooden stick,
and hits a small brass bowl. The sound of the bowl
rings around the tent, echoing, the women breathe
deeply into their bellies. Silence comes over the group
once more, before they disperse into the dark night.

Two weeks pass.

The day of the full moon arrives.

The girls who are coming of age are excited, but
nervous. They know that this is an honour and a
privilege to be invited to join this special red tent.

They wash their hair and put on beautiful flowing
white dresses. It feels almost like a wedding day.

Their mothers greet them at the door of the tent,
washing their hands with fragrant rose water, and
blessing their heads with it. The other women are
singing a hauntingly beautiful tune.

*The river she is flowing, rolling and flowing, the river she
is flowing down to the sea.*

The girls walk into the centre of the circle. Their
mothers join the circle of women around them.

One of the older women begins to tell a tale ...

THE GIFT OF THE MOON

By the silvery light of the full moon a little egg lay on a leaf.

And from it emerged a tiny caterpillar-girl.

The sweet caterpillar-child wriggled and played all day and ate and ate, and grew and grew. She watched the butterflies flying around her head—admiring their colours, but happy to be herself.

Until, one day, as the moon darkened, she began to feel a little strange, not quite herself any more. Hairs grew from her body. She wrapped herself up and hid, unsure what was happening in the darkness.

Inside the cocoon, magic was happening. Unseen. The magic of life itself.

The sweet caterpillar-girl that everyone knew and loved was changing. Until one day, she emerged, almost unrecognisable to her former self.

As she emerged, her body still taking shape, her wings drying in the wind, she was teased by the black bird.

"You're a freak, a flying worm! Your wings are weird!"

She tried to crawl back into her cocoon and hide, but she would not fit. Then she caught sight of the butterflies whom she had loved to watch as a caterpillar. They came to her and supported her as she leapt and learnt to fly. They danced around the sun, welcoming her.

Now she had wings to fly. She flew around in delight, comparing her beautiful wings to the petals which she passed. She was dizzy with delight.

And as the full moon shone once more, she found she was able to make babies of her own. She had her own miracle moons within her. They had been there all along ... she had just never known.

But as the moon darkened, she felt strange, not herself once more.

She remembered the days of the cocoon and wondered if she was about to change again? She felt more and more tired, and wondered if she was sick. She began to worry that she was going to die.

Old Grandmother Moon saw her tears and listened to her sad song.

"Dear child, do not cry—you are changing, but only on the inside this time.

"Do not fear! I will give you the gift of life. You can make babies at any full moon. But you need to cocoon yourself at dark moon, as your body remakes its magic. Then you can burst out again full of life, able to make love, life and beauty in the world once more."

The butterfly-woman agreed. And each dark moon time she cocooned herself quietly to rest, and when she was refreshed she emerged, with all her beauty to share.

So it is with you, dear one.

You carry within you the gift of life. As well as your beauty, you have your myriad creative gifts. But in order to give them to the world, each month, when the moon darkens and your blood begins to flow, you must allow yourself to rest, to dream and recharge, to listen to your inner world.

This is the sacred mystery of being a woman. This is the gift of the moon.

One of the women brings forth a beautiful white cake, iced like the full moon. They cut it and eat, and as they do they listen as one by one the women share their stories of their own entry into womanhood.

One tells of her bleeding which started when on a school canoeing trip. How this red river flowed out of her and she wanted her mother.

Another of how it started in class and showed through her skirt and everyone had pointed and laughed. How she put her jumper around her waist to hide it as she went to the toilet.

Another tells how she waited and waited, and all of her friends had their periods and she felt left out for being the only one without. She tells of her trip to the doctor where she discovered that her body was different, and that she would never bleed or have children. She speaks of how she learned to love her special body with its own unique gifts.

A woman with blonde hair and glasses, remembers that she was given a beautiful box by her mother filled with handmade pads, exotic bubble bath and moonstone earrings. Her parents took her out to dinner and made her feel special.

Another woman, much older, recalls the old fashioned pads that were bulky and uncomfortable, about how it was not the done thing to talk about their bodies, especially not 'down there'. And how her mother had put these pads on her bed, but never, ever said a word.

A small woman with short dark hair shares how she and her husband had taken their daughter outside and buried her first menstrual pad with her, returning her blood to the earth and giving thanks for her fertility and the fertility of the earth.

The women express the sadness that they felt at leaving behind childhood, and their excitement and confusion at becoming a woman. Their feelings of shock and surprise, or delighted expectation. The embarrassment of their mother or father. The reactions of their friends and siblings. So many stories, each so unique. Tears flow and laughter bubbles like a spring from the mountain.

Then one of their mothers stands to talk.

"It is time to share our first secret with you. It is **the secret of our blood.**

"Blood can mean danger. Blood can mean illness and even death.

"But the blood of your moon time means life and fertility. This is the blood of life, the blood of renewal.

"In the days before science and modern medicine women's monthly bleeding was a mystery—how could a woman bleed and yet not be ill? This was seen as a magical property held by women—to bleed and yet be well.

"You have a cradle of life within you, in your lower belly. Some call it the uterus, others the womb. This is where you grew within me.

"Just as the trees shed their leaves in the autumn to make way for new buds in spring, so too your womb loses its soft red lining every month if there is no baby to grow within you. This is your moon time, menstruation or period.

"This is a miracle of nature! **You are a miracle too.** Love your body, treat it with love and care. Just as we have done to it until now.

"Now is the time when you start to gently peel

yourself away from our care and become responsible for yourself and your choices. You are becoming your own woman!"

The girls were excited to have the first of the women's secrets shared with them. They felt relieved that in each woman's story they had found a little of their own truth. It made them feel like they were not alone.

Now the women's eyes turned to them. It was their turn to speak to the circle. The first stood, knees shaking, palms sweaty, to see the face of her mother and her friends looking up at her expectantly.

She began to tell her story of her first blood, only weeks before, her emotions still so fresh. It felt a little odd to be talking so intimately in front of all these women that she knew so well.

After she sat down, and her friend stood to speak, she understood the power of the circle and why it demanded such respect: **it requires great courage to speak the truth.**

The women embraced the girls, kissing them and whispering words of love in their ears.

"You are loved. You are strong, and beautiful and precious. We are here for you always, in good times and bad. We are so proud of you."

Then the women knelt beside them, massaging their feet and hands with scented oil, painting their nails with delicate colours and designs. They laid their hands on their bellies and blessed their wombs. Then gave each a special piece of jewellery: the first piece of jewellery that each had owned as a woman and one that would be treasured alongside engagement rings and wedding rings in the years ahead.

Then the girls were led out of the tent.

The full moon was high in the sky. They began to climb and climb the hill behind the tent. In the darkness they lost sight of the older women, until they didn't know which way to go. They felt lost and alone and scared in the darkness. Then they heard the voices of the women rising to meet them:

Follow the moon, follow your heart, keep your eyes on the moon and your feet on the path, and all will be well, my precious love, all will be well.

And then, around a dark and winding path, they reached the summit, a grassy dell bathed in bright moon light, with a heart of rose petals in the centre. They stood in the moonlight, exhilarated by their own power, soaking up the bright light. The women's voices were drawing closer, sparkling candles in their hands.

They embraced the girls in the moonlight and blessed them.

"Know that we love you and are here for you. Know that we understand, though we may be wearing older bodies, and the faces of mothers, aunts and friends. Yet we are all one, all part of the same experience, the same river of life and sacred female line."

They tied a red thread around each girl's wrist, connecting them to the group of women. "The red river flows through us all, the red thread connects us all." And then with a pair of golden scissors, the eldest woman cut the thread.

"We are connected but apart. We each must find our own path, follow our own bodies' wisdom.

"It was only the blink of an eye ago that we were in your shoes. We all travel the same spiral path in this life, though the steps of our dances are unique to us.

"And we know that there will be storms ahead of us, and know that at some stage you will need to break away. To cut the thread that binds us close. Know, dear child, that we hold the space for you to come back with love, as your own woman.

"You are our daughters, sisters and friends. We honour you for your future, for your growing beauty, your strength and intelligence, your wild creativity and growing confidence. We want to welcome you to the beginning of womanhood, this long and sacred journey of self-understanding and blossoming. Let us tell you the secret of the moon."

THE SECRET OF THE MOON

Each girl is born with a light inside her. A tiny, unique pin point of light. The potential for the woman she is growing into. With each birthday another candle is lit, and her light grows brighter.

The seasons begin to turn, spring turns into summer. New growth shoots—she grows upwards towards the sun and the moon, closer to their light. Her body sprouts its first signs of fertility—her breasts begin to round like the hills, her hips to sway like a river, her mound becomes forested, and secret dreams of womanhood begin to take her mind—of freedom, and love of boys or girls, and her potential. She grows and blossoms.

She learns that our bodies were born on this Earth, programmed by our genes and culture to be tied to the sun's daily rhythms for waking and sleeping, and to the moon for our menstrual cycle.

She learns that to let her light shine to its fullest glory, she must respect the rhythms of the Earth and the sky, the sun and the moon, the rhythm of her body.

She learns her lessons from the moon—when it is full,

so is she, she absorbs its energy and carries it with her—glowing from her face, her heart, her creations and words.

And when the moon is dark, she is quiet and rests. It teaches her that darkness is part of her—to be happy and healthy she must also go within, to recharge, reflect and rest.

Each month, throughout your life, the moon will lead you in and out—of yourself, of communing with those you love, of togetherness and apartness. Both are important. Watch her constant change and follow it. Grandmother Moon is a precious teacher for all women.

Many women find that their bleeding cycle is the same length as the moon's own cycle. And women who live together often find that their cycles match up, as their bodies communicate with each other. These are the mysteries of the moon.

We are not the only ones who are influenced by the moon—animals and plants are too. Corals spawn, wolves howl, many mammals go into labour and turtles lay eggs at the full moon.

People around the world—Pagans, Hindus, Muslims, Christians, Jews, native peoples all celebrate the full moon and its vibrant energies in different ways—from full moon parties on Thai beaches to Jewish family feasts. Many important fasts and feast days are rooted in the lunar calendar.

In the past most women bled when the moon was dark and released an egg at full moon. This was called a *White Moon Cycle*. A woman's energies are then in sync with the moon, helping her flow.

But things have changed fast in recent years. We don't live so close with other women any more, street lights outside and electric lights inside mean that our bodies are far less controlled by the moon's changing light levels. Artificial hormones and pollution in our water and food also affect our cycles. And so women find that they are feeling less connected to their bodies and their cycles. Less connected to the moon.

Nowadays women's cycles are staggered throughout the month. Some bleed at full moon, which is called a *Red Moon Cycle*, and many others are disconnected from the moon altogether, having much longer or shorter cycles.

Being disconnected from our bodies and nature's cycles, being stressed and always on the go leads to discomfort. Inside and out. Our bodies let us know that things aren't right by getting grumpy and tired and hurting. We need to rest when we bleed. But we live in a world which doesn't really understand this, and expects us to be the same every day: always bright and happy, nice and kind, always available and on the go.

Our women's cycles show us that we need 'down time' at certain times of the month. The moon guides us, by showing us her constantly changing face. She reminds us that we have our own inner rhythms that need to be respected far more than those of clocks and timetables. That is the only way to real health and happiness.

She is there to teach us, every day, every month, whenever we are willing to pay attention. Our menstruation is often called our *moon time*, because it connects our bodies with the cycles of the moon, and it reminds us to live according to moon time.

Phases of the moon

The moon is constantly changing in appearance—her shape and size determined by her position relative to the sun that illuminates her. Not only does she change in appearance, but also when she rises and sets. The moon has a cycle of approximately 29.5 days.

Full Moon

Full moons rise at sunset and set at dawn. They are energising—sometimes in a good way, and others creating agitation, making sleep and relaxation hard. Full moons are a time to harvest and sow, a time to entertain and celebrate, to work late and create wholeheartedly.

Each full moon has its own special name and character. For example the full moon which falls at some time in mid-August through to mid-September is called the *Harvest* moon—it tends to seem particularly golden and full, and was used to harvest by.

Waning moon

Waning means getting smaller. When the moon reaches its halfway point (the last quarter moon, which rises around midnight) there is a sense of balance, tension or transition. It continues getting smaller each night, until it is completely dark.

The dark moon or new moon

For a couple of days the moon is almost invisible—it is a time of darkness. The moon is in shadow and rises before dawn and sets with the sun. Many traditions use this as a time of inwardness, reflection, visioning and setting intentions for the month ahead. It is a time of new beginnings, a seeming pause in the darkness before its journey back to fullness again.

Waxing moon

The moon gets a little bigger and brighter each night, moving through the *crescent* moon—the moon of storybooks, the small sliver which speaks of hope, new life, magic. At halfway (the first quarter) again there is a sense of transition or balance, the moon is visible in the afternoon and sets in the evening.

Many cultures run on lunar calendars, but ours is solar. To learn more about the moon's phases, get yourself a calendar or diary with the lunar cycle in it. Look up at the sky every day, and mark the days of your cycle onto your calendar so you can see how your menstrual cycle and the phases of the moon interact.

OOO

Moon magic

The average menstrual cycle is 28 days long—which is about the same as the moon's cycle!

OOO

The most common menstrual pattern is to bleed on the dark moon and to ovulate at full moon.

OOO

The word *lunatic* was originally used to describe people who were strongly influenced by the full moon—we're all a bit lunatic really!

THE SECRETS OF OUR CYCLES

Part of learning the art of being a woman is learning to honour each element of our cycles and ourselves.

A cycle is the basic unit of life: birth, growth, transformation, decline and death, followed once again by birth. It is a circular, repeating journey. You see it in the beating of our hearts, the in and out of our breath, the seasons and the phases of the moon. Our menstrual cycles connect our female bodies directly to nature.

Your cycle takes you each month on a journey between the light and dark parts of yourself. Just as the moon travels from full light to darkness and back, every month. Part of learning the art of being a woman is learning to honour each element of our cycles and ourselves.

You can find yourself going from feeling loving, to feeling angry, from being creative to feeling numb. It can feel very confusing and bewildering to feel so out of control. This is where our women's wisdom comes in.

As we learn more about our cycles, and their unique patterns and the way that our moods change according to our cycles, then we feel less at sea and instead can swim with the tides of our bodies, rather than fight against them. This takes practice, and will be something that you are learning for years. But many women, who have not had the women's secrets shared with them, never know this. They never learn that the moon affects their cycles. Or that their mood changes are normal. Or how they can help themselves.

As you begin to sense your own rhythms you will gain confidence in yourself and dance to your own tune.

It is said that after your bleeding has finished you are the **maiden**—feeling young, fresh and energetic. When your egg is released you are like a **mother**—you can have a baby and you may feel nurturing and sociable. Then in the week before your period your mood can darken, you become a **sorceress** or **wild woman** who can turn anyone to stone who angers you. During your bleeding you are like an **old wise woman**—needing to rest more and full of insight if you allow yourself to follow your intuition.

Notice that these are the main stages of a woman's life—isn't it fascinating that your cycle takes you through these parts every month, so that you can experience each of them again and again?

THE GIFT OF THE CRAZY WOMAN

We do not talk very much about our dark sides.

But just as the moon is full at one time, at others it is dark. Just as it is with you. You are lightness and dark. Your dark side is symbolised by the Crazy Woman.

Long ago the Crazy Woman was depicted in the great myths and ancient holy temples. Her power was respected. She had the power to create life, but also to destroy it. Her dark side was respected as a crucial part of life. In different places she had different names: Kali, Medea, Durga and Hecate are just a few.

But as times changed, the stories changed. Her darkness was scorned. And she was turned into a witch, a feared out-cast. People were made suspicious of her.

Women were warned to only show their lightness. To be good and kind and beautiful. Their darkness, which is a crucial part of their power, was denied them. They were told it belonged to the devil.

But we all have a dark side, a shadow power. This is our anger, our fury our ability to storm and destroy.

This is the Crazy Woman—and she is in us all.

She is the dark side of a woman's loving and giving.

She is powerful! And that is her secret.

She is your power turned back on yourself and those you love. She is your shadow side with lessons to teach you about what you choose to hide away. She calls your deepest attention to that which you refuse to shine your light on.

She may terrify you, embarrass you, mess up your plans and your carefully done mascara! We fear her destructiveness inside ourselves and she is deeply threatening to our society. It can be pretty scary to feel her emerging. And scary for others to see.

She emerges when we are tired or overwhelmed. When we have given too much of ourselves away. When we refuse to say no. When people are too much in our space. When we are trying too hard to please others. When we are not being true to ourselves. She emerges when something we value is threatened or when our soul is at risk. She emerges as our blood time approaches.

"Listen to me! Care for me! Leave me alone!" She stamps and screams, yells and snaps. She emerges, raging, crying, shouting, threatening, hands shaking, face pale. Her message is true. But her ways of communicating are primitive and threatening.

So rather than let her out, we try to shut her up. Which only builds her up further. Never, ever shut a mad woman up in an attic or she will burn the house down!

So we need to find safe expression for the Crazy Woman. Copy down her words in your journal and heed them well! She is a wonderful teacher and will be with you your whole life long, teaching and guiding you.

We need to find balance in our lives so that she need not emerge too often or destructively. This is what all of us women are relearning every month. Sometimes we succeed and other times the Crazy Woman causes a lot of hurt and destruction around us with those we love.

Then we need to learn to ask for forgiveness of others when we have caused hurt. And forgive ourselves.

What have you learnt about the Crazy Woman—from your mother, grandmother, aunts, teachers, sisters or female friends? How have you experienced her in yourself?

THE GIFT OF PREPARATION

The appearance of your first blood (called your *menarche* or *first moon*) can be quite a shock and surprise. Especially if no one has told you about it!

One of the gifts we want to give you is that of preparation. Of seeing the signs that tell you that your period is approaching and being prepared so that you know what is happening to you and how to respond. This takes the worry and stress out of it.

Nobody knows exactly when your periods are going to start—not you, not your mother or your doctor. But the age your mother started is a good clue to when you might ... so ask her if you can.

There are other clues too, including:

  o Getting taller—most girls grow about 10cm or more in the year before they start their periods, you will be almost your full adult height when you start bleeding.

  o Your breasts growing. They start to bud first, and then 2–3 years after first budding your periods will come.

o Changing discharge coming from your vagina which might be white or yellow—this starts 6–18 months before your periods.

o Pubic hair appearing on your genitals and under your arms—periods normally come 1–2 years after your pubic hair.

o Your hips and thighs starting to change shape as you put down fat. You need to have enough body fat to start menstruation, so please, please do not try to diet or exercise it away. It is normal, natural and a necessary part of having a woman's body.

o Hair and skin starting to get greasier.

o A few spots on your face or back.

o An aching belly or lower back.

o Stronger feelings and turbulent emotions.

Girls' periods start on average at 12 years old, usually between 11–14. But that is just an average, and you are unique! Some girls start at 8 and others at 18, and some never get them at all. If you don't have yours yet, but your friend does, don't panic or think there's something wrong. It's not a competition! Talk to someone you trust.

The age of starting your cycles depends on lots of different factors, including whether you have enough body fat. **It's really important to know this, as there can be lots of pressure on girls to be really skinny and not eat properly.** Some girls and women have naturally super slim bodies. But if you try to force your body to be what it is not, it will not be able to grow or cycle as it should.

You may have noticed that your friends are shifting and changing too—some faster, some slower. We all have our own inner timetables that cannot be forced or changed. We start our periods at different times, have different length cycles, have babies at different times (or not at all), and finish our monthly bleeding when we are older at different times, just as we will die at different times. We are each of us unique. Our journey throughout our lives is accepting our bodies in their uniqueness.

But for you, whenever your time comes, it marks the beginning of your fertility. Your first period officially marks your transition from child to young woman.

It signals the point where you are able to carry a new life within your body. This is a big deal—right?

It will still be years before you decide to become a mother, or you may never choose to. But the ability to create and carry new life is truly magical. And something that only women can do.

If you don't know how babies are made, now is a

good time to put down this book, and ask an adult you trust. It's really important that someone you love explains to you the magic of life. And I will not be explaining it here, because it is a big topic, and one that different people like to explain at different times. I am assuming that you know the basics of reproduction. So if you don't, go and ask!

I don't want to assume that you know anything about periods. You might have covered them in a science class, or perhaps at home.

Let's make sure we all have a solid, shared understanding. And I guarantee that everyone will learn something! Even I did when I was writing this, and I've been bleeding for over 20 years!

From the age of about 12 to 51, unless you are pregnant or on the pill, every single day of your life as a woman will be somewhere on the menstrual cycle.

Throughout the month your body is in constant change, responding to the changing levels of hormones (natural body chemicals). This is your menstrual cycle.

Some of the many changes include:

○ changes in body temperature

○ the texture and acidity of your vagina and womb

○ the size of your breasts

○ how you see and hear

○ how you feel and respond to pain

○ your moods and emotions

○ how your body holds water

○ even your heart rate!

This is why it is so important to learn to listen to your body throughout your cycle and know what "normal" feels and looks like for you.

When you understand that your body is always changing, but that the rhythm of these changes follows a regular pattern, then you can begin to live within your body's cycles rather than fighting them. Then you know that it is perfectly OK to go to bed early some days, because that is what your body needs. And that at other times you will be full of energy.

It is when we don't do this and carry on as normal every day, ignoring our body's signals and symptoms that we start to have problems like pain, fainting or exhaustion.

So how can you best prepare yourself for your first bleeding?

○ Get a couple of sanitary towels to have in your bag and bathroom.

○ Read a little bit of this book so that you feel a little more confident and aware.

○ Ask questions so that you feel confident and prepared.

○ Start thinking about how you would like to celebrate becoming a young woman.

○○○

Our incredible bodies

Because of earlier puberty, lower breastfeeding rates, better nutrition, longer life spans and fewer pregnancies, women today have more periods than ever before! So understanding your cycle is even more important, as you're going to have about 450 periods in your life time!

I will be describing a typical 28-day cycle—but remember, your cycle might be a lot longer, or a bit shorter than this (mine is currently only 25 days) ... so this is only a general guide.

Bleeding time/menstruations (Days 1–5)

○ The first day of bleeding is referred to by doctors as **Day 1** of your cycle.

○ Bleeding usually lasts 4–6 days, getting lighter in the final couple of days until you return to your clear flow of discharge.

○ Your uterus (or womb) is about a third larger than its non-menstrual size, rich and swollen with blood.

○ The bleeding happens because the rich womb lining which had been waiting to carry and feed a baby is not needed as your egg that month has not been fertilized.

○ It flows down through your vagina and is red or brown in colour.

○ It is often a deep red to begin with and sometimes has small clots (or lumps) in.

○ Only an egg-cup full of blood is lost, but it looks like a lot more!

○ Blood is red because of iron—so we have to be sure to keep our iron levels up during our cycles by eating iron rich foods or taking supplements. If you are very pale and often very tired or dizzy, you might be low in iron.

○ A missed period doesn't automatically mean you're pregnant. If you haven't had sex, then you can't be! Maybe you're tired, stressed or have you been ill?

Pre-ovulation (Days 6–13)

○ *Pre* means 'before', *ovulation* means 'egg making'. So pre-ovulation is the time before the egg is released.

○ A hormone called oestrogen increases in your body.

○ This gets your body ready to develop and release an egg, and also prepares your womb and breasts for possibly getting pregnant.

○ You have had your eggs since you were in your mother's womb! You have many thousands but only a few hundred will ever mature and be released, and fewer than ten will ever be fertilised!

O You may have clear discharge from your vagina.

O You will probably feel much more lively and energetic.

Ovulation (around day 14)

O At ovulation time (around day 12–16) usually just one egg is released from an ovary (where they are stored) into one of your fallopian tubes, which look a little like cows horns or the branches of a tree.

O The egg is the size of the head of a pin.

O If a sperm from a man's penis reaches it now it may well be fertilized and begin the nine month transformation into a baby.

O You will notice a change in your vaginal discharge around this time. You will most likely feel very wet, and your underwear will be damp. It can often feel like you have just got your period because you are so wet. You might choose to wear a panty liner to protect your underwear.

○ Ovulation discharge is clear and stretchy like egg white. If you put it between your fingers it will stretch 5–10cm! This makes it easier for sperm to swim in and fertilise the egg.

○ You will most likely feel sexier and have excited dreams and thoughts. This is perfectly normal and natural.

○ You need to be extra careful of pregnancy now if you are having sex. But it is really, really important that you do not rush into intercourse. Just because your body can now make babies, it doesn't mean that it should! Growing up is a time of massive change, and it is really important that you get really comfortable in your own body before sharing it with others. Hormones and friends may be pushing you to have boyfriends, but there is no rush.

Pre-menstrual

○ The pre-menstrual stage can last for up to a week before bleeding starts.

○ This change in hormones can lead to pre-menstrual syndrome (PMS for short—more on this later) symptoms including anger, moodiness, bloating and achiness. It gets stronger as you get older, especially after having children.

○ Your vaginal discharge becomes thicker, often cloud white or yellow, more blobby or lumpy.

○ Most women have a second window of sexual excitement either just before or towards the end of menstruation. This is completely normal.

○ You need much more dreaming sleep from day 25 of your cycle, through the first three days of your bleeding.

○ You may have memorable dreams at this time which communicate important ideas or messages to you. They might be very powerful or scary. They often have important messages.

Many women have regular cycles of around 28 days, though others might have cycles of varying lengths (14–40 days), and periods of varying lengths (3–7 days). When your periods are first starting in your teens, and when they finish in your late forties or early fifties, they may well be quite irregular as they get into their own rhythm.

What is most important is that you know what 'normal' is for you. Some women naturally have shorter or longer cycles their whole lives, however if:

- O your periods are very irregular

- O you have a lot of mid-cycle spotting, (little bits of bleeding throughout the month)

- O your period is very light (pale pink and watery)

- O or it is extremely heavy

- O it contains lots of clots

- O your PMS symptoms are really severe

then do be sure to go and see your doctor. Irregular cycles over a long while often mean there is another health problem that might need to be looked at.

You need to be aware that many medical doctors may suggest going on the contraceptive pill to deal with all sort of period related issues including:

- O period pain

- O heavy bleeding

- O acne

O irregular periods

In truth you are much too young to have to even think about the pill, but many doctors use it as their treatment of choice for all sorts of period problems. So this is why I am mentioning it here.

The pill is a cocktail of artificial hormones which affects your menstrual cycle by tricking your body into thinking it is pregnant. It is also used as a contraceptive (to stop women getting pregnant).

When women take the contraceptive pill, the bleeding that they experience every month is not a real period but simply a 'withdrawal bleed'. So the whole time that you are on the pill your body is not following your natural menstrual cycle, which as we have seen, is important for your health.

My moon time in my teens was hard. Not only did I have the mood swings of teenage girlhood and PMS, but my period pains were so bad that I would often faint in the first couple of days of menstruation. I would be writhing in agony, often on bed rest with a hot water bottle and as many pain killers as I could safely take.

I was a high achiever, with full busy days at school. The mentality around periods was that they got you off swimming, but that was it—carry on regardless, they shouldn't have any impact on you. And so I tried to do that for years.

The doctor prescribed me the strong painkiller Ponstan at first, which had little effect. He told me that period pain would get better after I had children, which was, we both agreed, a very long way off. He then placed me on the contraceptive pill. I was 16 and proud to be on the pill. Looking back now that makes me feel angry that there was no other way of helping me to deal with this.

I felt sad, depressed, as though I was floating below the surface of life. I didn't feel like myself on the pill, but because I couldn't point to any definite symptoms, or explain what that really meant, no one would take me seriously. No one told me it was because I was cut off from my own rhythms. No one said that this is quite a normal feeling ... on the pill.

Think long and hard before going on the pill, it may seem handy and even cool, but it has a lot of short and long-term side effects on your body that you need to be aware of.

It is an extremely useful drug in certain cases, but is very over-prescribed by over-worked doctors who have little else to offer. The side effects are not properly explained to most young women and they include:

- mineral depletion in your bones leading to brittle bones in later life

○ imbalanced emotions and sex-drive

○ depression

○ putting on weight

○ possible fertility problems when you are older

○ doubled risk of breast and ovarian cancer if you take it under the age of 20

○ possible blood clots in your legs

For a fuller understanding of the effects of the pill, if it is ever recommended to you, do read *The Pill: Are you sure it's for you?* by Jane Bennett and Alexandra Pope.

I highly recommend trying some of the natural remedies for painful periods that I share later as they do not have this nasty list of side effects.

CELEBRATING THE FIRST MOON

The chances are you will never forget your first period, and even when you are an old lady you will remember where you were and who you told first.

This is my story …

The first time I found out about periods I was nine and at school. Just before leaving junior school each girl was issued with a little pocket-sized booklet entitled *Personally Yours*. I still remember the cover, a fuzzy image of a reclining girl with a blonde bob, pink jumper and jeans. We were intrigued. We took them outside at lunch break and three of us girlfriends lay on our backs, legs up to the ceiling in a concrete crawling tunnel in the playing field, and devoured this new information. We were fascinated.

For me it was to be three years before I experienced it for myself at twelve. I remember being in my flute lesson. I felt muddle-headed, clumsy, frustrated, and very vulnerable. I cried and cried. My poor teacher, was as kind and understanding as he could be, I was obviously just having a "bad day". I went to the toilet after the lesson. And there, to my amazement was lots of red blood on the toilet paper. I felt excited— knowing that this was a big deal for me, for my life. A shift, a change had happened. School was over for the day. But it was a boarding school so I would not be seeing any of my family until the weekend. It felt momentous. I needed to share that I was changed. I grabbed my best friend, and we went outside. We walked in the gardens and I told her. It felt so right to share it with a female friend, and to do it out in nature.

But being in boarding school also had its downsides. I felt a deep shame. I didn't want anyone else to know that I had my period. So I used to cough really loudly when I opened the crinkly sanitary towel wrapper, or wait till the toilet was flushing! I spent ages scrubbing leaks from my underwear, so that the nuns who washed our clothes would not see my blood.

Only trusted friends knew when I was "on". We used to watch each other's backs—literally! In the summer term we wore white and blue striped skirts which showed leaks very easily. It was a sisterhood. We had a special code word, "P", which then, for reasons unknown to me, became "Mr P". Then because my father was Mr P, we called our periods "Stephen", after my dad! It seems very strange to me know that our periods had a man's name, though we didn't see that at the time!

My mother cried when I told her. And I told my stepmother too. They were both lovely and so good with any practical questions I had, there was no awkwardness. I swore my stepmother to secrecy—she was, after all, the sisterhood. But at some point, my father figured out that I had gotten my period, and was hurt that I had not told him. I got a five page letter from him expressing this. What business is my blood of yours? I wondered. I felt vulnerable for having my privacy, my secrecy, broken, and by a man.

And so it continues to this day. My trusted sisterhood knows where I am in my cycle. It feels like a sacred secret that they understand, because they've got it too!

In traditional cultures, girls who are becoming women would be celebrated by their whole tribes, a little like the red tent celebration you read about at the start of the book. I am sorry to say that these are still not common place in our own culture, which I feel is sad. Because YOU deserve to be celebrated.

You might want to talk to your friends about creating one together. Or ask a special woman in your life to organize one to mark your menarche, or first blood. You might choose to have it on the day of your first bleeding, in the month of your first cycle, or in a year or so when you feel more ready …

Even if you have had your period for a couple of years, it doesn't mean you have to miss out on a menarche celebration. I know of women who have celebrated their entry into womanhood when they were in their thirties, because that was the first opportunity they got!

When you do it, or how you do it, is not as important as doing it—doing something—whatever feels right and comfortable to you, to mark the change from girl to woman.

Maybe you don't want to have a big event, but would prefer to do something special privately by yourself, or with a special friend.

If so some of these ideas might take your fancy!

- O write a poem or do a painting

- O get your ears pierced

- O or a new haircut

- O bake a cake

- O get a piece of jewellery—maybe a ring or bracelet to mark the occasion

- O pick yourself a beautiful bunch of flowers

- O get a special moon journal or moon dial

- O have a special dinner

- O have a make-over from a special girl or woman

Creating ceremony

We are used to creating ceremonies in our culture … birthdays, Christmas, weddings and funerals. But there are many, many important life passages that go completely unmarked. Part of our reweaving of women's culture is a claiming of these rites of passage as important and finding ways to mark them which are meaningful to us.

You do not need to be religious, or even spiritual to create and enjoy ceremony. Think of a birthday party— this is one of the most common rituals in our culture— we send out invitations, set a pretty table, make a cake, light candles, blow them out, our friends sing us a song, give us gifts and cards which are meaningful to us, wish us well for the year ahead, perhaps make speeches and then share food with us. A birthday party contains all the elements of the ceremonies I mention in this book.

So even if you are new to ceremony, or a little uncomfortable with the idea, chances are you have celebrated many, big and small, in your lifetime already. And whilst it is easier to follow the well-worn traditional rituals of birthday parties, because we (and our guests) know what is expected of us, making new celebrations such as to mark menarche or first blood is exciting—as we are creating them fully in our own images—with no expectations.

If you are excited at the thought of having a bigger celebration, here is a step by step guide for creating your own menarche celebration ...

- O Invite a circle of women to celebrate with you—your mother, sisters, friends ... you set the date, time and venue!

- O Decorate the space beautifully—red and white flowers, candles, inspiring pictures, drapes, incense—make it feel special and sacred.

- O Perhaps dress in red or white to celebrate bleeding and fertility.

- O Have a special welcome—perhaps walking under branches, or over scattered rose petals. Have your hands and feet washed with rose water and your hair brushed.

- O Maybe ask someone to be your moon mother, or godmother if you don't already have one— what older woman would you like to be your mentor as you grow up?

○ Read a poem, prayer, blessing myth, story or passage from an empowering women's book (see the resources section at the back of this book for lots of great books).

○ Get your guests to tell the stories of their first bleeding, how it felt, what it meant, how it was received.

○ Have your hands or belly painted in henna, or your fingernails painted.

○ Join hands and sing or just stand quietly together.

○ Create a necklace or bracelet together which you can wear to remember this day.

○ Get everyone to bring you special gifts.

○ Have a book where your guests can write in some special words for you.

○ Bake a full moon cake, like in the story at the beginning of this book.

○ Light a candle of blessing.

○ Eat together afterwards—you might even choose all red food!

THE GIFT OF CHARTING

Your first cycles might differ a lot in length. You might have 40 days between your first and second periods, followed by a couple of shorter cycles as your body matures.

But once you have started to have regular periods, it really helps to know where you are in your cycle. Then you will know when to expect your period, (and importantly when to have sanitary towels in your bag and be wearing dark underwear!) when you might feel very emotional and need more rest, and later when you need to be super-careful not to make a baby by accident!

Keeping track of your cycle

The simplest way of keeping track of your cycle is in a diary. Create a special symbol or code—perhaps a star or a red dot or a spiral and put this on the date your flow starts. Then use another symbol for the last day of your flow.

You can count forward 28 days (or however long your cycle usually is) and put another symbol, perhaps a question mark on the date that your next period is due.

As women we don't very often take the time to note down the changes in our bodies, or reflect on them. But they have so much to teach us. Why don't you write a few notes in your journal every day for a month to see how your cycle affects you on a daily basis? You can then read it back day by day during your next cycle to see how similar your internal experience of each month is.

Let me share with you the ups and downs of a real cycle, so that you can see the changes of moods and energy throughout the menstrual cycle. If you have already started your periods, you might recognise yourself and your own patterns which previously had gone unnoticed. Or you might have noticed these changes in your mother, but not realised they were part of a regular cycle.

(Remember that in talking about cycles, day one is the first day of bleeding.)

Day one

I feel big and heavy, my belly feels massive and my boobs are a bit achy. I feel like I am in a dreamy bubble, my brain is moving slowly.

For the past couple of days I have known that my moon time is approaching. I know from the sky: the moon has gone and the nights are really dark. I know because I wanted to be alone with my thoughts, to write in my journal and not talk to anyone.

Before I would have ignored these signals until I lost my temper and shouted at my family. Now I know I can just say I need to be by myself for a while. I head up to bed early with a hot water bottle.

Day two

I am tired and slow. I take it easy and rest as much as I can. My bleeding is heavy.

Days three and four

I am less tired as my bleeding gets lighter, I still feel quiet.

Day five

With my bleeding gone I feel the need to purify, to cleanse. I always have a bath on this day, to wash away the smell and feel of menstruation. It is a time for scrubbing off dead skin and old feelings, to break fresh and clean into the new cycle. I don't like having baths during my bleeding so it always feels like a real treat to have one. I luxuriate with a rose candle, bubble bath and steam rising up.

Days six to eight

My libido starts to rise. I feel buzzy and alive. I want to be close and affectionate, where only three days ago I desired nothing more than to be alone and untouched.

Days nine to twelve

My energy is soaring. This is the fertile time, when all my children were conceived. It is a time for creativity—with body and soul. I have so many projects that I want to start right now!

Days thirteen and fourteen

Full moon is here and with it my ovulation—I feel deeply connected to the brightness of the moon. I also feel a little crampy at this time of the month. I head outside and dance in the moonlight, and give thanks for all I have.

Day seventeen

Day seventeen always takes me by surprise—I find myself snappy and impatient, and so, so tired. It must be the day that my hormones shift.

Days eighteen to twenty four

I notice my energy levels starting to lessen—I am between the worlds, neither ovulatory nor premenstrual. Some days I feel fine, others I am cranky.

Days twenty five to twenty seven

A tireder, heavier energy emerges, I feel sluggish, and everything is an effort. I would really just like to curl up like a cat in a cosy chair in front of a roaring fire, and not be bothered. I cry my eyes out in front of a soppy TV program and growl about everybody's imperfections. I snap impatiently at my family and then burst into tears once again. I feel yucky and hate myself and everyone else.

Day twenty eight

I need to be nurtured, and I know I don't want a bath. I get this sense of not wanting to be in water just approaching my period. I need warming food, a blanket round my shoulders, to curl up in a seat and soak up gentle goodness. And chocolate, of course chocolate! My absolute **need** for chocolate reaches a crescendo in the week before my period. It is so strong. And so necessary: dark, comforting warmth that soothes me.

This is my retreat time. It is a time for woolly socks, cosy jumpers, a good book, crying at girly films, and did I mention chocolate?

THE GIFT OF SELF-CARE

Learning to really care for yourself takes years! It sounds silly because it seems so obvious. But often we prioritise everything other than ourselves. We put our friends, socialising, school, hobbies and sport ahead of the basic things in life that create health: rest, eating well and other basics. Looking after yourself becomes really important when you have your menstrual cycle, especially in the few days before your period and whilst you are bleeding. Your body is doing extra work, and needs plenty of rest and care to support it.

Here are a number of ways to care for yourself, shared with me by women around the world:

- ○ In my grandmother's words: SIMPLIFY, SIMPLIFY, SIMPLIFY! This is your mantra for a better moon time.

- ○ Eat nutritiously and keep your blood sugar levels stable.

- ○ Don't do too much physical activity—no running a marathon when your period's due!

- A short, gentle walk or bike ride outside does you the world of good to reconnect with yourself and nature and get the energy moving.

- Have you discovered yoga?

- Keep your clothing comfortable—especially if you get bloated or chilly at this time.

- Do something to make yourself look and feel beautiful—wear a special necklace, a lovely scent, a pretty top ...

- Make no major decisions!

- Take time every day for yourself.

- Try to get to bed in good time. Your need for dreaming sleep increases in the pre-menstrual period and lack of it causes PMS.

- Do everything you can to make yourself feel good and loved. Try repeating positive affirmations to yourself: I love and accept my body exactly the way it is. I love and approve of myself.

- Scream into a pillow.

- Take ten conscious breaths.

- Have some special quiet time with a friend.

○ Let your hair down, your tears out and your feelings be heard.

○ Write in your journal.

○ Get a punch bag and beat it!

○ Do not try to change your world or those around you just because you are angry and frustrated.

○ Bathe yourself in the positivity of others if you are feeling dark—uplifting books, films, blogs ...

○ Listen to music that lifts you.

○ Do some receiving from your family: get a massage, a shoulder rub, a hug ...

○ Snuggle up with a hot water bottle or castor oil pack.

○ Brew up a pot of herbal tea.

○ Go to the health food store and get some supplements for yourself.

○ Eat chocolate!

○ Have you tried acupuncture, cranio-sacral therapy, reiki, reflexology, or chiropractic treatment?

- O Start a dream journal.

- O Be gentle and loving with yourself. Always.

THE GIFT OF REST

As you have learnt by now it is really important to rest before and during your period. Your body will let you know it needs to rest as it will feel tireder than usual. So listen to it. Don't ignore it!

Our culture does not have any real days of rest, as our ancestors did with the Sabbath. Nor do we have permission to 'take it easy' during our moon time from the outside world, as the Native Americans and ancient Canaanite women did in their moon lodges and red tents. Often when we rest all sorts of uncomfortable feelings can come up (and comments get made). We might feel:

- O lazy

- O like we ought to be doing something

- O that we're wasting time

- O guilty

- O bored

Your moon time is the time when you are feeling

tiredest, slowest. Your body needs rest, and your mind needs quiet. Creating a retreat space for yourself allows you to honour your body's natural energy cycle. It is a time when your intuition is strongest. Intuition is a sense of knowing that we cannot explain. Some people call it gut feeling or instinct. It is usually not logical. It is an important part of your own wisdom and it tends to get stronger at your moon time.

Many women refer to the quiet time they need during moon time as "retreating to their cave"—think dark, quiet, and being left alone.

In practical terms this means picking the right time of day, and a place that you can shut a door to or share with other girls and women who are celebrating their moon time too.

Here are some ways you can create your very own private retreat space for your moon time . . .

O **Shut the door, draw the curtains**, turn off your computer and phone.

O Make your space feel **womb-like, safe and contained**.

O Have **gentle lighting**. This helps you to shift into a more relaxed, peaceful frame of mind and helps you to feel like you have had a real rest even if you don't sleep.

○ Perhaps you might like to **use essential oils** to relax you.

○ Make a **hot water bottle** and put it on your belly if it is aching. You could use a hot pad or castor oil pack instead.

○ **Get yourself a big glass of water or herbal tea.**

○ **Breathe deep into your belly.**

○ If it helps you, **do a guided meditation** (perhaps the happy womb visualisation on www.thehappywomb.com).

Journaling

I'm sure you probably already have a diary or journal where you write down your private thoughts and feelings. I started writing journals when I was 11 and I have been doing them ever since. They are a great way to vent your feelings and reflect on your life.

Dream journaling

Our moon time is often a time of powerful dreams which can stay with us through the day. They can often be dark, scary dreams around our blood time. Sometimes we might get powerful messages or ideas from them. By keeping a journal we record the wisdom of our dreams and begin to understand our own personal dream language.

Moon letters

A dear friend and I wrote moon letters over the course of a year. Every moon time we would sit and write a handwritten letter—we shared our dreams, visions for the month ahead, reflections, quotes from books, poems we had written. These were our way into reconnecting with our own cycles, sharing our wisdom and insight and learning to take time out. It really deepened our friendship sharing something so private.

Self-care regime

Now is a great time to enjoy the self-care practices that I shared earlier—perhaps do a face mask or manicure, gently massage your belly with some scented oil. Take time to brush your hair or moisturise your skin— nurture and care for your body.

Meditation

Meditation is a practice of still being, where we slow down our thoughts and fully relax our minds and bodies. There are many different types of meditation that you can learn in classes, but meditation needn't be a formal practice. Simply slowing your mind whilst breathing into your belly, gazing at the moon out of the window, or listening to the wind whistling or gentle music—all of these bring us into a state where our mind can let go of being in control.

Intuitive practices

Tap into your stronger intuition in whatever way you can. The special women in your life might teach you some of their practices.

Reading

Now is the time to immerse yourself in a book which feeds your soul—perhaps something spiritual or meaningful to you as a female. In your menstrual phase you are especially sensitive, so stay away from horror or thrillers which can overload you emotionally.

Creative doodling/imaginative painting/collage

Another really great way to further understand your changing moods and feelings through your cycle is through your creativity.

You don't need to be a 'good artist' to have a go! Your pictures don't need to be 'perfect', as long as they mean something to YOU.

Whatever you choose to do, take this opportunity to fill yourself full to the brim with love, inspiration, gentleness and beauty.

THE GIFT OF HERBS

For years women were the healers of their communities. And even now, the chances are if you've hurt yourself or feel unwell, the first person you will go to is your mother, who will often know of a remedy for you.

Doctors and prescription medicines have a really important place in healing our bodies. But they are not the only way. There are lots of wonderful natural remedies to support your body in its cycles.

Herbs are part of the traditional wise woman approach to health. Cultures around the world use the healing powers of plants to help support the female body and soul from Chinese herbs (often given alongside acupuncture), to Ayurveda (alongside yoga), Native American and traditional European wise woman herbalism. Herbs were our first medicines. And many prescription medicines still come from them!

Herbs tend to be much gentler than medical drugs, and work with the body, rather than simply hiding symptoms. They tend to have few unwanted side effects. However, they are still very powerful and we need to have respect for herbs, in just the same way as we do for pharmaceutical medicines.

Be sure to work with someone as you learn to take care of your body. Talk to your parent or guardian, go to a health food store and ask their advice, perhaps go to see an alternative therapist. Learn from their knowledge and experience.

Remember I am not a trained herbalist, and I do not know your unique body—so be sure to seek further advice.

Key herbs for moon time

These can be bought loose or as tea bags from a health food shop. Or you can use fresh or dried leaves that you have grown yourself.

You can use tinctures in water, or even tablets or brew herbs together to make tea. Use them individually or mix a few different herbs for your own signature brew!

- O Shatavari—the Queen of Herbs for women. It is used in Ayurveda (traditional Indian medicine) to lighten menstrual bleeding and generally support the female hormonal system.

- O Lemon Balm (Melissa)—to soothe and relax. Lovely as a refreshing tea.

○ Evening Primrose—great for relieving PMS symptoms, taken ten days before bleeding starts. Especially effective for easing tender breasts.

○ Cramp Bark—great for easing cramps in the womb, hence the name!

○ Red Raspberry Leaf—tones the uterus and helps if you're feeling queasy.

○ Feverfew—for migraine and headaches (can be eaten fresh in salads and sandwiches).

○ Nettle—good for iron. Often girls starting their period can get low on iron (anaemic).

○ Chamomile—to soothe, relax and help sleep.

○ Shepherd's Purse—to ease excessively heavy bleeding.

○ Motherwort—good to ease cramping. It has been used by women in labour for centuries

Flower remedies

These can be taken as drops on the tongue or sipped in a glass of water. They are made by soaking the plants in brandy to extract their 'essences'. They are really great for emotional balance—you may have come across Rescue Remedy before, which is a blend of five flower essences and is great for shock or panic.

O Holly—for when you're feeling prickly!

O Oak—for strength.

O Impatiens—for impatient feelings.

Essential Oils

These oils are made from the crushed flowers or leaves of plants and can be used in an oil burner, on a hanky or your pillow, for massage, steam inhalation or in a bath. They are very strong and should always be used diluted in a base oil (like sweet almond oil) if applied direct to the skin.

O Rose—a very sensual, feminine scent.
Also good for soothing anger.

O Geranium—sweet smelling.
Good for depression and stress.

O Juniper—great for reducing bloating and swelling.

O Chamomile—calming and great to help you sleep.

- Lavender—calming, good for migraines and headaches. Great to help you sleep. Put a couple of drops on your pillow.

- Neroli—good for soothing, weepiness and depression.

- Mandarin/Orange—uplifting!

- Clary Sage—a powerful scent. Brings clarity to the mind.

THE GIFT OF FOOD

How do you feel about food? Do you love to eat or do you worry about putting on weight? Do you nourish yourself with good things or pig out on junk food that makes you feel great at first, and then sick? Do you enjoy regular nutritious meals or do you not eat until you really have to, or maybe you live off snacks ... ?

Sometimes we eat instead of feeling or expressing our emotions. When we feel upset we can eat lots of junk food to try and make ourselves feel better. Or we stuff ourselves with sugar to boost our energy levels rather than resting.

As women we need to have a healthy relationship with food and what we fuel our bodies with, because it is our food that rebuilds our bodies every day and keeps us healthy.

One of the simplest ways to care for yourself is by eating well, especially in the days before your period.

    O   Make sure you drink lots of water, fresh juice and herbal tea. Avoid fizzy drinks and caffeine.

○ Water or fresh apple juice with fresh lemon juice, grated garlic and ginger is a powerful tonic for your body.

○ Many women swear by green smoothies to boost energy, especially during moon time. Add a large handful of leafy greens (spinach, kale, lettuce and perhaps some spirulina) to your normal smoothie base of banana and juice, blend and serve.

○ Consider taking supplements of B vitamins, especially B6 and B12, iron, zinc and magnesium, especially leading up to menstruation and if you are vegan or vegetarian.

○ Zinc relieves cramps. It can be found in dark green vegetables, wild plants, seaweeds and nuts.

○ Eat lots of green leafy vegetables, red meat and dried fruits for iron to ensure you are not anaemic.

○ High protein foods such as meat, dairy, seeds, fish and chocolate are great for lifting your mood.

○ The caffeine and sugar in chocolate lift your spirits—but they can give you a headache, so watch out!

○ Cut back on sugar, caffeine and processed foods if you find this improves PMS symptoms.

○ Many women find that they have added cravings for simple carbohydrates (potatoes, bread, cake and sugar) and meat approaching their moon time.

○ Some suggest that eating red meat at this time can make your bleeding heavier, so you might want to experiment and see what works for you.

In everything you eat—honour yourself.
In every rest you take—honour yourself.
In how you spend your time—honour yourself.
In the people you spend your time with—honour yourself.
In nourishing your body and soul with love and mindful awareness, you learn to truly honour everyone and everything that your life touches.

YOUR QUESTIONS ANSWERED

We all have them—big questions and little ones. Questions that burn a hole in our hearts, and seem impossible to ask, and practical ones that we might feel silly not to know. Questions are how we learn.

Come close, my sweet. Ask me your questions. Do not be shy. Whisper them in my ear, and I will do my best to answer. Ask the women you love and trust ... they are longing to help you find your answers.

I have period pain what can I do?

The first thing is to rest. Sit down or lie down. Then, if you can, get a hot water bottle or hot pad and put it on your belly. Taking basic painkillers should help as well.

If you struggle with cramps regularly, have a look at the herbal healing section with an adult for herbal supplements that you can take to ease the pain.

I feel sad and miserable, is this normal?

There are times during every woman's cycle when she feels down. Everything feels wrong. You might feel miserable for seemingly no reason. You might feel very under-confident and down on yourself, like everything you do is lame. You might burst into tears at the moment's notice, and find that your feelings get hurt very easily. This is completely normal in the pre-menstrual phase of your period. Let yourself cry—with a good friend or in private—it is a great release and will help you to feel clearer and calmer. It's an odd thing, but having a good cry often makes us feel better.

Be sure to take it really easy on yourself. Relax with a movie or a good book, talk to a good friend, write in your journal or draw. Remember that this too will pass, but in the moment it feels like it will last forever.

If it goes on and on for more than a week, be sure to let someone know, you might be struggling with bigger stresses, maybe even depression. The most important thing is to reach out to people who love you. You are not alone.

Why am I so angry?

Bursts of anger and impatience can flare up in your

pre-menstrual time. You might find everyone and everything irritating. You might be cross at yourself because you're being clumsy, forgetful or don't have enough energy. Shouting is a great release, but try not to do it AT people, as angry words can be very hurtful, and you can feel very bad later for lashing out. The same with physical violence—it can be a great release of tension—but don't hurt people. Hit a pillow or a punch bag, play a hard game of tennis or squash, take up martial arts ... It is OK to feel angry. Often women feel embarrassed about their anger—but it is a perfectly natural emotion.

What do I use to soak up my blood?

When women bleed they use something to collect or absorb the blood flow so that it doesn't make a mess in their clothes, or on the floor or seats. In the past, women would use moss or old rags to soak it up. In the red tent they would squat over straw which would be used to fertilise the fields. Menstrual blood is great for helping plants to grow.

Nowadays there are disposable sanitary products which most women buy from a shop. There is a huge range of products that you can use for periods now. These are some of them with their pluses and minuses to help you make an informed decision. Each woman and girl has to find what works best for her at this part of her life. And it is also important to bear in mind what impact your decisions make on the Earth.

Sanitary towels/pads

There are lots of brands of sanitary towels in any chemist and supermarket. They are very thin nowadays and come in lots of sizes—night time ones are very long to prevent leakage. Some have wings to go round the outside of your underwear and help them to stick even better and prevent leakage—but this does mean that when you are getting changed people will see them.

Disposable pads

Made of thin absorbent material, backed with sticky plastic, you stick them into your normal underwear like a plaster—they are a bit like a small nappy! Do NOT flush them down the toilet, but dispose of them in a bin. Some are scented.

Pluses:

- o Can be bought anywhere and quite cheap.

- o Stick easily to your underwear—like a plaster.

- o Comfortable.

Minuses:

- These are disposable and cause big waste disposal problems globally, millions are floating in the seas and cause danger to wildlife.

- Perfumed ones may cause irritation.

- The plastic covering can cause rubbing and chaffing on some people.

Washable cloth pads

Usually made from soft cotton or flannel with varying layers of absorbent material inside. They usually have wings that fasten with a popper underneath.

Pluses:

- They are reusable and so much more environmentally friendly.

- Soft and comfortable.

- Many women say that their flow is less heavy wearing these.

- You can make them yourself.

Minuses:

- You need to wash and dry them.

○ Not quite as handy on holidays or trips or if you are out all day, as you have to carry the used ones around with you.

○ Can be expensive to buy to begin with, but once bought they will last many years.

Tampons

Tampons are a compressed type of cotton wool with a string tied to one end that you place inside your vagina to absorb your flow.

Pluses:

○ Cheap and easily available.

○ Good for wearing tight clothing, doing sport, swimming and gymnastics.

○ Your vulva stays clean—it makes your period seem invisible and odourless.

Minuses:

○ You shouldn't use them for the first six months of having a period or when your flow is lighter.

○ It takes time to get used to putting them in, and can be uncomfortable if you get them at the wrong angle, and sometimes if you are a virgin.

○ Must be changed regularly.

○ Environmentally damaging—there are millions of used tampons polluting our waterways.

○ Can cause Toxic Shock Syndrome, a rare but very dangerous condition which can be fatal.

Moon cups

Like a tampon but made of silicone, a moon cup catches the blood in your vagina. You simply empty the cup into the toilet and then reinsert it.

Pluses:

○ They can be washed in a sink quickly and easily.

○ Clean and easy to use.

Minuses:

○ It takes time to get used to putting it in. Can be trickier in your first years of menstruation.

○ About £20 ($25)—but you only need one!

○ Not so easy to use in public toilets where the sinks are public and not in the cubicle.

Sponges

Sponges are also placed inside your vagina as a natural alternative to tampons.

Pluses:

○ Natural and safer than tampons.

○ Cheaper than moon cups.

○ Easier to insert than moon cups.

Minuses:

○ Can be messy/tricky to use in public toilets.

○ Need to be replaced every few months.

Whatever you choose to use, it also it helps to have:

○ Dark underwear.

○ Dark or red towels.

○ Darker clothes so that you are not worrying about stains.

How do I deal with my blood?

Firstly just keep wiping yourself until there is almost no blood on the paper.

Then unwrap the sanitary pad/towel (if it is in a wrapper) so the sticky back is showing.

Stick the pad onto your underwear, being sure it is in the centre of the gusset.

If it has wings, remove the backing from them and fold them underneath your underwear.

You will probably need to change your pad every time you go to the toilet whilst your flow is heavy.

Do not flush them down the toilet. Wrap the used pad in the wrapper of the new one and dispose of it in the sanitary bin beside the toilet. Or take it in your pocket or bag to a suitable rubbish bin.

Always have a spare sanitary pad in your bag.

If you find yourself without one you can ask another woman or friend, and public bathrooms often have pads for sale. Or if you really don't have anything, roll up a big wad of toilet paper and put it into your underwear. Get a pad as soon as you can!

What do I do at night?

You might want to use a bigger, night time towel for

when you go to bed. There are a couple of reasons for this. Firstly you will not be changing it as frequently, and secondly they are longer, so that they do not leak.

You may want to sleep on a dark towel if you bleed very heavily.

If you get blood on your clothes or sheets it is best to soak them as soon as possible so that it doesn't stain. There are lots of stain removers for sale that you can use, but often just soap and water and a quick scrub in the sink before you put it in the laundry does the trick. Soaking blood stains in milk is a traditional cleaning solution.

It feels good to wash yourself every day. This helps to keep your vulva clean, to prevent odour and help you to feel fresh and comfortable. You can do this standing at a sink, in a bidet, or in the shower.

It helps to have a dark coloured bath towel to dry yourself with so that you are not worrying about blood stains on towels.

The same goes for underwear—dark knickers are much easier during moon time.

What colour should menstrual blood be?

The blood starts out as a deep red, changing to a brown or pink towards the end of your flow. There may be small clots or little flecks in it. This is completely normal.

Will anyone know I have my period?

It is unlikely that anyone will be able to tell you have your period. Although you may notice that you smell a little different, it is not obvious to others. The biggest giveaway is your mood swings in the few days before.

What if I leak?

This is a big worry for many girls. The first thing is once you have your periods to keep track of them in your diary so you know when you're expecting it. If you do leak, don't panic, wrap a sweater round your waist and change your clothes as soon as you can.

How do I put a tampon in?

With tampons (and moon cups and sponges) practice makes perfect. It helps if you wait for a few months until your flow is heavier and more regular. Then ask a woman you trust for guidance—you need to be able to relax your vaginal muscles well to insert a tampon.

I think I am bleeding too much ...

Your flow can seem extremely heavy on the first 2–3 days, and when you first get your period you might be surprised by the amount of blood that there seems to be. When you are first starting your periods they can be extremely heavy—earlier in the book I shared herbal and nutritional advice for helping to lighten your flow naturally.

What is discharge? How does it change through the month?

Vaginal discharge is an important part of your female health. Every woman has it. It keeps your vagina moist and helps keep it clean. The discharge changes throughout your cycle. Starting slightly cloudy, becoming clear and stretchy when you ovulate and getting thicker and yellow or white pre-menstrually.

If it is very white and itchy you may have a common infection called thrush or candida, and need to go to the pharmacist or doctor to get a simple medication to clear it up.

My belly feels tender and swollen. I feel fat!

We can all feel fat, blobby, and generally unattractive pre-menstrually. It might just be a feeling, but you also might have water retention which actually means that your clothes feel tighter and uncomfortable. Your womb almost doubles in size when you are bleeding, so it is natural to feel your stomach is fuller and more rounded.

See the herbal section of this book for herbs that can help with water retention.

Can I swim/shower/have a bath?

You can absolutely have a shower, bath or swim when you have your period. The flow tends to stop when you are in water, but a little may still come out. However any blood that is on your pubic hair or vulva will come off in the water, so do clean yourself before you go swimming.

Many women choose to use a tampon or moon cup to catch their flow so that they don't have to worry about any blood flow. If you are going to be on the beach all day in a swimming costume then you will need to use a tampon or cup.

I tend to choose not to swim or have a bath during my

bleeding time—I just don't feel like it and stick to showers. But I really enjoy my first bath when my flow has stopped.

What is PMS?

PMS (pre-menstrual syndrome) or PMT (pre-menstrual tension) happens in the week or so before your bleeding starts and often continues for the first couple of days of your flow.

It can include any (or all) of the following symptoms:

○ a bloated belly and water retention

○ tearfulness

○ being snappy, angry, short-tempered, impatient

○ cramping

○ lower back ache

○ dizziness, nausea, fainting

○ migraine or headaches

○ forgetfulness, brain fog or difficulty making decisions

○ spots, greasy skin and hair

○ tender, lumpy, larger breasts

It has been said that our modern world, with its busyness and stresses is a perfect way to create PMS for women.

For some women these symptoms may start over a week before their period comes and may continue throughout their bleeding time. This is no small matter if two weeks out of every month are filled with physical and emotional suffering.

Have you noticed older women's changing moods? Ask them how they deal with PMS and what works for them.

THE GIFT OF YOUR SISTERS

Do you have good friends who feel like sisters? You may already have found some special sisters who will walk beside you in life, honouring and celebrating your journey with you. One thing is sure, you will meet many more along the way as you move through your teenage years and on into adulthood. Take time to build strong relationships with your friends, to have fun together and listen to each other. Be there for each other in good times and bad.

Girls and women can sometimes be pretty mean to each other. We can feel threatened by each other—and be bitchy and hurtful, especially in our teenage years, when we're all feeling insecure. But there is another way of being together—which makes us all more powerful: sisterhood. In sisterhood there is no need for jealousy, because we know that there is no competition: we are all special, we are all unique, there is space for all of us, and all of our voices, our stories have value and deserve to be heard. It truly doesn't matter what you look like, how old or young you are or what you can do: you are valuable. We each have gifts to share, lessons to learn, and experience which can help others.

To close the circle of this book, your older sisters, women of many years life-experience, want to share what they wish they knew when they stepped over from girlhood to womanhood:

"I wish that I knew that it was all going to be OK."

"I wish that I knew that I was beautiful—even though I felt fat, and untrendy and spotty at the time, photographs of me then show a beautiful, slim girl."

"I wish that I knew I didn't have to be tough all the time. That it was OK to be sad, to be quiet, to not have all the answers, and have people care for me."

"I wish I knew that I had a whole world of like-minded friends out there to meet when I was stuck in my small, boring, narrow minded school—that it would just take us a few years to find each other."

"I wish I knew that I really wasn't alone. That although girls can be bitchy and mean, they are also wonderful support and that talking things through with them is the greatest gift in the world."

"I wish I knew that too much sugar made everything

much worse—my mood swings, weight, energy levels."

"I wish I knew that there really was nothing to be embarrassed about, that we are all the same underneath—and all a little bit different too."

"I spent a long time waiting for others to accept me—I wish I knew earlier that what I needed to do was accept myself, and then the acceptance of others didn't matter very much at all."

"Courage is not just bungee-jumping or driving fast, but speaking your truth quietly, and living your life the way you want to."

"To not listen to those who wanted to bring me down—it was their own fear, their own anger, their own problem, not mine."

"To trust my intuition."

"To take time to rest."

"I have learnt that tears are not a sign of weakness but of strong emotion. They are holy water."

"Wherever I go, whatever I do, I'll always be there—so I might as well start being my own best friend!"

PARTING WORDS

As we reach the end of our time together, you will have had many of your questions answered and hopefully feel more excited about your changing body and moon time. But you may still have more. Take time to share them with an older woman that you trust.

Thank you for your company on this journey.

I want you to know that you can:

- be proud of yourself as a girl and woman

- know that you are beautiful, awesome, incredible, just exactly as you are

- learn to trust that your body holds immense power and wisdom

- be true to yourself

- commit to self-care

- know that you are loved. Completely. Just for being you. Shine your light bright, do what you love, learn to follow your body's wisdom.

This is the path of becoming a woman.
These are our secrets.

Blessings to you, bright, beautiful girl.

Lucy Pearce, Cork, Ireland, May 2015.

RESOURCES

As you grow up you may want to find more books which support you on your journey into womanhood and help you understand the magic of your body. Most of the books below will be of interest to girls aged 15 and over.

Online resources

www.thehappywomb.com for moon dials, books and articles on womanhood

www.moontimes.co.uk for moon bracelets, dials, diaries and calendars

Do be aware that a number of other online "information" sites are actually promotional sites run by the manufacturers of sanitary products or supplements. Their information is, therefore, biased, as they are trying to sell you something.

Books for girls

Menarche: A Journey into Womanhood—Rachael Hertogs

A Blessing not a Curse: A mother daughter guide to the transition from child to woman—Jane Bennett

A Diva's Guide to Getting Your First Period—DeAnna L'am with gloriously creative and bright illustrations by Jessica Jarman-Hayes

Moon Mother, Moon Daughter—Janet Lucy & Terri Allison

Puberty Girl—Shushann Movsessian

The Thundering Years: Rituals and Sacred Wisdom for Teens—Julie Tallard Johnson

The Seven Sacred Rites of Menarche—Kristi Meisenbach Boylan

First Moon—Maureen Theresa Smith

Becoming Peers—DeAnna L'am

Becoming a Woman: A Guide for Girls Approaching Menstruation—Jane Hardwicke Collings

A Time To Celebrate: A Celebration of a Girl's First Menstrual Period—Joan Morais

Books for women

Moon Time: harness the ever-changing energy of your menstrual cycle—Lucy H Pearce

Red Moon: Understanding and using the creative sexual and spiritual gifts of the menstrual cycle—Miranda Gray

The Red Tent—Anita Diamant

Thirteen Moons—Rachael Hertogs

Herbal Healing for Women—Rosemary Gladstar

Neal's Yard Natural Remedies—Susan Curtis

The Beauty Myth—Naomi Wolf

Women's Bodies, Women's Wisdom—Dr Christiane Northrup

The Pill: Are you sure it's for you?—Jane Bennett and Alexandra Pope

Read my Lips: A Complete Guide to the Vagina and Vulva—Debbie Herbenick & Vanessa Schick

Circle of Stones—Judith Duerk

73 Lessons Every Goddess Must Know—Goddess Leonie Dawson

Women Who Run with the Wolves—Clarissa Pinkola Estes

Resources

The Vagina Monologues—Eve Ensler

She Walks in Beauty—A Woman's Journey Through Poems—selected by Caroline Kennedy

Herstory—free e-book of women's history available from www.moonsong.com.au

ABOUT THE AUTHOR

Lucy Pearce is a passionate teacher and writer on the topic of womancraft—the art and craft of being a woman that your mother never taught you. She is mama of two daughters and a son and lives in a little pink house in the village of her birth in County Cork, Ireland.

Together with her husband, she runs a publishing imprint, Womancraft Publishing, creating life-changing, paradigm-shifting books by women, for women. They are champions of new technology, building strong collaborative, creative partnerships, human-friendly working practices and fair profit sharing. They offer editorial and mentoring services through their company Lucent Word.

A former contributing editor at *Juno* magazine, Lucy wrote her popular column, Dreaming Aloud for the magazine, for almost five years.

She blogs at Dreaming Aloud.net, where she muses on creativity, motherhood, mindfulness and living philosophy.

Her website, The Happy Womb.com is a repository of empowering resources for women.

Lucy is the author of four books:

O *Moon Time: harness the ever-changing energy of your menstrual cycle*, has been labelled 'life-changing' by women around the world. It is the best-selling book in its field.

O Her girl's version *Reaching for the Moon* is a soulful guide to the menstrual cycle for girls aged 9–14 has been heaped with praise from parents and daughters around the world.

O *The Rainbow Way: Cultivating Creativity in the Midst of Motherhood*, was a number one Amazon bestseller in a number of categories in the US and UK. Featuring the voices of over 50 creative mothers including: Jennifer Louden, Julie Daley, Pam England and Leonie Dawson it has been credited for kick-starting numerous creative careers and saving lives.

O *Moods of Motherhood: the inner journey of mothering,* gives voice to the often nebulous, unspoken tumble of emotions that motherhood evokes. It has been received with deep gratitude for its honest exploration of maternal experience.

Her work has received great acclaim from her own creative heroines, as well as women around the world. Her guest posts have been featured on Rhythm of the Home, Tiny Buddha, Wild Sister, The Big Lunch and TreeSisters.

Lucy has also become known for her vibrant visual art, particularly her lost archetypes of the feminine series. Her work has been commissioned for magazines, book covers and family portraits.

Contact her at lucy@thehappywomb.com

Womancraft Publishing

Life-changing, paradigm-shifting books
by women, for women.

Visit us at: www.womancraftpublishing.com
where you can sign up to the mailing list and receive
samples of our forthcoming titles before anyone else.

Follow us on Facebook: Womancraft Publishing
Follow on Twitter: @WomanCraftBooks

Please do leave a review of this book on Amazon or
Goodreads.